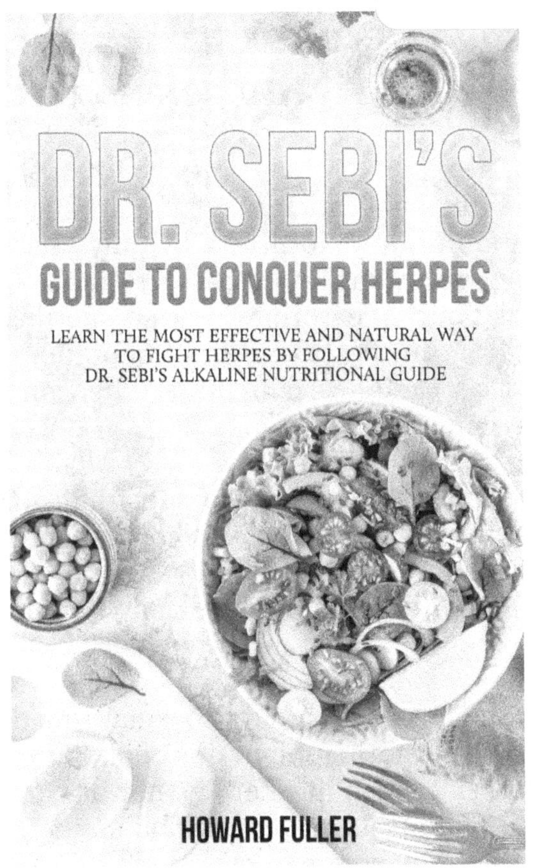

Dr. Sebi's Guide to Conquer Herpes

Learn the Most Effective and Natural Way to Fight Herpes By Following Dr. Sebi's Alkaline Nutritional Guide

Table of Content

Introduction

Herpes is a viral disease. It is a family of several diseases called herpesviruses. These are the viruses that cause cold sores, genital sores, chicken pox, and shingles. Herpes infections can be caused by eight different types of herpesviruses.

There are two types of herpes infections. One is genital herpes. This is called Herpesvirus hominis (HVH) and it affects the mucous membranes in the area of the genitals and buttocks. The other type is a cold sore or fever blister called Herpesvirus type 1 or HV1.

Herpes is generally transmitted through oral-genital contact, but it can be transmitted through any skin contact with an infected site. When it is transmitted from mother to child at birth, it can cause serious illness or death in an infant. It can also be transmitted to a newborn from anyone else who has been exposed to the virus, even if they do not show any signs of an infection.

Herpes simplex virus two (HSV-2) can cause genital sores that eventually go away on their own, but they will most likely recur and be painful for a short period of time before they heal up again. Symptoms of herpes simplex are painful blisters or sores in the genital area of men and women which break open, ooze and become crusty before healing over about 2 weeks time without leaving any scars. If you have been suffering from one form of herpes for some time, you may be more susceptible to the other type.

Herpes simplex is a chronic condition that can stay hidden. That is why it is so important to know your status so that you can take the right precautions to prevent transmission of the virus.

Herpes is a virus and, as with any other virus, it can be successfully treated and cured. And the best news is that Dr. Sebi has found a way to cure it without the use of pharmaceutical drugs or medications.

Dr. Sebi is a world-renowned herbalist, author, and healer. He is also a medical anthropologist and was born in Honduras. His primary goal is to teach people how to cure themselves of their ailments through holistic methods. Dr. Sebi has found that the way to do this is to eat the right foods, take vitamins, and take herbs. His philosophy is that if your body is healthy, it will be able to fight off any disease that comes its way.

In this book on Herpes, we will learn how Dr. Sebi became interested in helping people with herpes and how he became aware of the problem of herpes when he came in contact with many people who were suffering from it. Some of these people were his relatives and friends and others were patients for whom he was prescribing herbs. We will also learn about his recommended natural remedies and cures for different types of herpes, including genital herpes, chicken pox, shingles, febrile disease (fever blisters), cold sores (oral herpes), and glandular fever (infectious mononucleosis).

After reading this book, you should be able to:

1.Identify the types of herpes and the stages of each type of herpes infection.

2.Learn how to prevent future herpes outbreaks by following Dr. Sebi's recommendations for diet and herbal supplements.

3.Learn how daily vitamin intake can help your body fight off even an active herpes outbreak.

4.Learn what your herbal and nutritional treatment options are for an active herpes outbreak.

Without proper nutrition, herbs, and vitamins, it is impossible to cure herpes. The most effective way to treat herpes is by using both a natural holistic approach and other pharmaceuticals or medications that you may already be taking.

Chapter 1

The Definition of the Herpes Virus

Most people have heard of or had experience with the herpes virus. Many people are infected with herpes, but very few know the true definition of it. This chapter is for anyone who wants to read about the latest discoveries and information about the herpes virus and how it relates to HIV.

What is Herpes?

Herpes viruses are enveloped, double-stranded DNA viruses belonging to the family Herpesviridae. Herpes simplex viruses (HSV) are the causative agents of herpes simplex virus type 1 (HSV-1) and herpes simplex virus type 2 (HSV-2), commonly known as, respectively, oral and genital herpes. The family also includes varicella zoster virus, which causes chickenpox.

The human herpes viruses (HHV) are a large family of DNA viruses that infect humans and many other animal species. The family includes several important pathogens causing diseases such as mononucleosis, chickenpox, shingles and cold sores. The HHVs belong to the order Herpesvirales, family Herpesviridae, subfamily Alphaherpesvirinae .

The HHVs constitute three distinct subfamilies (alpha, beta and gamma-herpesviridae). Each subfamily contains multiple herpes viruses with distinct replication strategies, antigenic properties and clinical symptoms. All human herpes viruses establish lifelong latent infections in individual hosts through integration of their DNA into a specific site on host chromosome 8 long arm (8q). In addition to this common feature for all HHVs, there are significant differences in both disease course and epidemiology between the different human viral infections caused by this family.

Herpes Simplex Virus Type 1 (HSV-1) is the causative agent of herpes simplex virus and causes cold sores or fever blisters around the mouth or lips. HSV-1 infection can also lead to infection of the eye, which can cause conjunctivitis (pink eye), keratitis (inflammation of the cornea), and keratoconjunctivitis (inflammation of both cornea and conjunctiva). HSV-1 may also become active in the genital area, causing herpes genitalis . In such cases, it is likely to spread from the genitals to cause herpes labialis . The virus is transmitted through skin contact, usually by kissing or sexual contact with an infected person. It can also be passed from mother to baby before birth. It is a highly contagious virus that can remain in active state for life in a person who has never had an outbreak.

Herpes Simplex Virus Type 2 (HSV-2) is the causative agent of genital herpes . Although HSV-2 infection has been traditionally associated with female genital tract infections, it is now known that about 40% of all new genital infections worldwide are caused by HSV-2.

The History of Herpes

The herpes virus is a very ancient and incurable disease. It has been known to mankind for more than 5500 years. The medical profession has known about herpes since about 1880.

Since the mid-30s, the medical profession has done nothing to cure or even prevent herpes. Herpes simplex virus 1 (HSV-1) is one of two types of viruses that cause herpes infections in humans. HSV-1 most commonly causes oral herpes, which can result in cold sores around the mouth and on the face, lips, nose, and eyes. In rare cases, HSV-1 may also cause genital herpes. HSV-2 most commonly causes genital herpes. However, it can also cause infections of the skin or mucous membranes in other parts of the body.

The Lifecycle of Herpes

There are 8 phases to the life cycle of a virus:

Phase 1: Attachment

The virus binds to the surface of the cell and disables its interferon response.

Phase 2: Penetration (by fusion or endocytosis)

The virus enters the host cell. Fusion is used by enveloped viruses and endocytosis is used by non-enveloped viruses. The virus may enter either by binding to receptors, which are found on the surface of the host cell, or by rupturing the membrane of the host cell. Fusion and endocytosis both result in viral entry into the host cell cytoplasm. The virus may remain uncoated within endosomes or may be released from endosomes into the cytoplasm.

Phase 3: Release of viral genome (uncoating)

In this phase, the viral capsid disassembles and releases its genome into the cytoplasm of the host cell, where it can attach to a cellular ribosome for translation. In some viruses, notably poliovirus, this phase begins during penetration before entry into the cytoplasm has occurred; in such cases it is known as 'reversible uncoating'. The viral genome can remain in a free form within the host's cytoplasm, or can be integrated into the host cell's DNA.

Phase 4: Translation of viral genome (replication)

The viral genome, once it has entered the cytoplasm, is translated by the host cell ribosomes into polypeptides. As polypeptides assemble into a virus particle, they may be transported back out of the cytoplasm by an export motor protein or they may remain in the cytoplasm.

Phase 5: Virion assembly and release from host cell

Naked viruses assemble at the cell membrane, whereas viruses with an envelope assemble within endosomes. Enveloped viruses acquire their lipid envelope when budding from the plasma membrane, while non-enveloped viruses acquire their envelope after nucleocapsid assembly. Virions are extruded through pores in the host cell membrane and are released from the host cell shortly afterwards. Following release from its host cell, a virus may infect other cells or remain latent within its original target for long periods of time. Herpes simplex is a virus of this type; it can cause latent infection within neurons and neural ganglia. In such cases it remains dormant until triggered by certain events such as stress or immune deficiency.

Phase 6: Replication of viral genome (reproduction)

In this phase, the virus uses its own synthetic machinery to translate and assemble viral proteins and nucleic acids. In many cases, viruses transcribe and translate their genomes to produce complementary RNA strands (sense or antisense). These complementary RNA strands are then used as a template for producing viral progeny nucleic acid strands (viral mRNA, complementary DNA etc.). Viruses that use RNA as their genome have the additional step of producing a DNA intermediate during replication. The DNA is then transcribed into mRNA, and the mRNA is translated to produce more viral proteins. The newly produced virus particles then assemble and release from infected cells.

Phase 7: Assembly and release of new virus particles (propagation)

This phase is the same as the previous phase, except that it involves the production of new virus particles.

Phase 8: Death of host cell (apoptosis)

The host cell dies and ruptures as a result of steps taken by the virus during its life cycle.

Why Herpes is so Common

In the United States, HSV-2 infection affects about one out of every six individuals aged 14–49 years. Studies show that genital herpes is common in the United States. It is estimated that more than one out of every six people aged 14 to 49 years in this country has genital herpes infection. In addition, it is believed that more than 90% of those infected are unaware that they have the virus because they are asymptomatic or have very mild symptoms. HSV-2 often causes no symptoms, but when it does, they can be mistaken for another skin condition such as a yeast infection or jock itch.

HSV-1 and HSV-2 are different but closely related viruses. The viruses are so closely related that antibodies against HSV-1 will sometimes react to HSV-2 infection and vice versa . It is believed that up to 90 percent of the adult US population has already been exposed to HSV -1, although most people experience no symptoms or have only mild symptoms from the virus . About 40 percent of people become infected with HSV -2 during their lifetime.

The herpes virus is passed from person to person through direct skin-to-skin contact. HSV-2 is spread through direct contact with an infected person's genitals, buttocks, or mouth. It is less likely to spread when there are no visible sores or symptoms. HSV-1 is most often spread through oral-to-oral contact; however, it can also be spread through other types of skin-to-skin contact .

The herpes virus can be shed from a person's body even when they have no symptoms of having the infection. Although the amount of time that the virus is present in a person's body varies from person to person, it can be difficult to know exactly when someone has become infected because people are often unaware that they have been exposed.

It is important for people with HSV infection to understand that although they may not always experience symptoms of a genital herpes episode, they are still capable of passing on the virus to their sex partners. It is also possible for people who think they may have herpes not to actually have the infection and for people who think that they are not infected with herpes to actually have it.

Conventional Herpes Treatment

Before we get into the natural and holistic treatments that are recommended by Dr. Sebi, let's look at some of the conventional treatments that are prescribed for herpes.

According to Dr. Sebi, most doctors only treat the symptoms of the virus and not the virus itself. They are trained in dealing with symptoms and not causes. **The drugs that are prescribed for herpes include:**

1.Acyclovir

Acyclovir is a prescription drug that is used for the treatment of herpes, genital warts and shingles. It is available in generic form and it is also marketed under various brand names. Physicians also use it for the treatment of chickenpox and acute herpes zoster infections in patients who are over the age of 13.

2.Famciclovir

Famciclovir is an antiviral drug that is used for the treatment of herpes simplex virus infections. It works by slowing down the growth and multiplication of the virus. It stops the spread of infection and can prevent new outbreaks from happening. The dosage frequency as recommended by doctors is twice a day for 5-10 days depending on your condition. Your doctor may also prescribe it to be taken for one week after an outbreak occurs until all of your symptoms have cleared up.

3.Valacyclovir

Valacyclovir is a prodrug medication that must be converted into acyclovir in order to be effective in fighting herpes infections. It works by suppressing viral replication and preventing new outbreaks from occurring. The recommended dosage frequency as prescribed by doctors is twice a day for 5-10 days depending on your condition or as directed by your physician. There are also other drugs that can be prescribed by doctors such as famciclovir, valaciclovir, penciclovir and others but these are only used in severe cases.

Most often, doctors only treat the symptoms of herpes and not the actual cause of the virus. They may prescribe acyclovir (generic or brand name) to be taken orally or as a cream or ointment.

Chapter 2

Identifying the Symptoms of Herpes and How Its Spread

In this chapter, you will be introduced to the symptoms of herpes. We will also learn how Herpes commonly spreads and how to mitigate the spread of the infection. Before we get into the treatment that is recommended by Dr. Sebi, let us discuss the symptoms of herpes and understand how it is transmitted.

By understanding the symptoms of herpes, we will be able to identify people who are infected and take steps to prevent ourselves from getting infected. Also, when we are infected, we will know how to manage the symptoms and prevent ourselves from spreading the virus to other people, while undergoing Dr. Sebi's treatment.

How Herpes is transmitted

There are many ways that herpes can be transmitted, including contact with the infected area, contact with the fluid that flows from the infected area during an outbreak, contact with the fluids on a towel that is in direct contact with the infected area, contact with a person's saliva, and contact with an object or surface that has been contaminated by an infected person's body fluids.

Let's take a look at the most common ways that herpes is transmitted:

1.Contact with the infected area

This is the most common way that herpes is transmitted. When a person with herpes has an outbreak, there will be fluids that flow from the infected area. If you come into contact with these fluids and are not wearing any protective gear, you can get infected.

If you touch an area of your body that is infected with herpes and then touch your mouth or nose, you can get infected. This can also happen if someone gives you a hug or kiss without wearing protective gear on their lips or mouth. It can even happen when your lips or mouth come into contact with a towel, pillowcase, cup, or utensil that has been used by someone who has an active outbreak of herpes.

2.Exposure to the infected partner's fluids

The herpes virus is found in the fluids of an infected person. This is how you can get herpes even when your partner does not have an active outbreak. If your partner has herpes and he or she comes into contact with his or her own fluids and then begins to touch you, he or she can transfer the herpes virus to you.

This is why it is so important for a person who has herpes to never touch his or her own face without first washing his or her hands. This will help prevent the spread of the virus from taking place.

3.Sexual contact with a person who has an active outbreak

Another common way that herpes is transmitted is if you have sexual intercourse with someone who has an active outbreak. The reason for this is because the fluids from your partner's genitals can come into contact with your genitals and cause you to become infected. If the infection spreads, it can cause serious health problems such as sores on your mouth, vagina, penis, or anus.

4.Pregnant women can pass on herpes to their child

Another way that herpes is transmitted is if a pregnant woman has herpes and passes the infection to her unborn child. This can happen when she is near the end of her pregnancy. The baby can become infected with herpes if the mother has an active outbreak around the time that she gives birth. The baby can also become infected if the mother has an active outbreak during delivery.

What are the common symptoms of Herpes?

The most common symptoms of herpes are blisters, ulcers, and sores in the mouth or on the genitals. Genital herpes can be spread through sexual contact.

Genital herpes is a sexually transmitted disease (STD) caused by the herpes simplex virus (HSV). The virus causes painful genital sores and can lead to genital lesions that last for weeks.

If you have a cold sore, you should avoid oral sex or oral contact with your partners genitals. If you have herpes, using a condom may help prevent spreading your infection to other people.

Some people who have genital herpes are aware of their infection because they have experienced symptoms. Many others do not know they are infected because they have no symptoms or they mistake their symptoms for another condition or no condition at all (asymptomatic). In fact, most individuals with HSV-2 infection are unaware of their infection. They do not know that they ever had an active outbreak and do not realize that they may still be infected with the virus and may still be contagious to others .

Complications of Herpes: Herpes can cause complications both inside and outside the mouth . One of these complications is called Bell's palsy which is a facial nerve paralysis. Another is called herpes keratitis which is an eye infection caused by the herpes virus . The most serious complication of herpes is a rare occurrence of a brain infection known as herpes encephalitis .

It is important for you to be aware that the primary risk of acquiring genital HSV-1 or HSV-2 infection is not having sex (abstinence) but rather the frequency of your sexual relationships. There are several other factors, however, that can increase your risk of contracting genital herpes including oral-genital sex with someone who has a cold sore, being younger than 30 years old, having multiple sexual partners, and having a weakened immune system due to illness or medication.

Symptoms of Herpes Type 1

1.Blisters or sores appear on the mouth, lips or face.

This is the most common symptom of herpes. Even though it is not a visible sign, the virus can be transmitted from one person to another during kissing or through oral sex.

2.A "tingling" sensation in the area of the skin where an outbreak will occur.

This symptom indicates that an outbreak is about to happen in that particular area, and you should avoid contact with anyone who may have contracted the virus. If you are able to predict this symptom, there are some natural remedies that may prevent or shorten an outbreak of herpes.

3.Sensation of skin irritation in the area where an outbreak will occur.

This symptom can be either a warning sign of an impending outbreak or a symptom that one is coming. If you feel skin irritation, this may be an indication that your body is trying to rid itself of the virus in some way. Oftentimes people with this symptom experience relief from their symptoms after exercising.

4.Pain and itching in the area where an outbreak will occur.

This may also be a sign that someone who has contracted the herpes virus is trying to get rid of it naturally through the body's natural healing processes. Itching and pain are a warning sign that there are active viruses on or near your skin. This indicates that you should avoid sexual contact with anyone who has not been tested.

5.A slight fever.

This may also be a symptom of the body's attempts to rid itself of the herpes virus, but it may also be a sign that you have contracted the virus. This is why it is so important to take a herpes test as soon as possible after any type of sexual contact with someone who has contracted the virus. Getting tested sooner rather than later will help you know if you have contracted or if you are about to contract this highly contagious and potentially life-threatening disease.

6.Tiredness, aches and pains in the area where an outbreak will occur.

This is another sign that your body is trying to rid itself of the herpes virus before an outbreak occurs, but like all other warning signs it may indicate that you have already been infected with this disease or that you are about to be infected with it at any moment in time. This is why it is so important to get tested after having any type of sexual contact with someone who has contracted or may have herpes simplex 1 or 2. Early diagnosis can help prevent the spread of this disease.

Symptoms of Herpes Type 2

1.A burning or itching sensation in the genital area

When this condition becomes acute, the itching or burning sensation in the genital area is usually accompanied by a tingling or aching pain. This is followed by redness and swelling of the skin.

2.Lesion, blisters and bleeding sores

These are some of the symptoms you will experience when herpes type 2 is in its acute stage. The lesions appear as red bumps that are either raised or flat to the touch. Sometimes, these lesions may be accompanied by open sores. The blisters will burst open after three to seven days, forming unsightly ulcers with a yellowish base referred to as "dead skin". After this stage, the ulcer heals but it leaves behind an unsightly scar on the affected areas which may last for weeks or months before disappearing completely.

3.Fatigue and severe muscle pains

Herpes type 2 is known to cause fatigue and severe muscle pains such as muscle aches and respiratory problems when it is in its acute stage. This condition makes your body tired and exhausted while at the same time, inhibiting your ability to breathe freely when you sleep at night. This stage of herpes type 2 may also be accompanied by excessive sweating and clumsiness.

4.Abnormal bleeding from the genitals

It is not uncommon for people suffering from herpes type 2 to experience abnormal bleeding especially after sexual intercourse. This may be accompanied by the swelling of the genitals and even nausea. If left untreated, it can cause death. But, when treated early enough, herpes type 2 would not kill you. In fact, it can be cured completely with herbal remedies like Dr Sebi's Herpes Cure for Herpes Type 2.

5.Swollen lymph nodes in the groin area

Herpes type 2 is known to cause swollen lymph nodes in the genital area which could be located near the groin region or lower abdomen. The swollen lymph nodes are usually painless but they can get painful when you touch them or when you urinate. The swelling of these lymph nodes may also cause fever and feeling of weakness and exhaustion among people with herpes type 2 infection.

6.Pain in the joints

Herpes type 2 is known to cause pain and swelling in the joints especially those that are close to the genital areas. The joints may get swollen and become painful but they can be treated with herbal remedies like Dr Sebi's Herpes Cure for Herpes Type 2.

7.Skin rashes

Herpes type 2 is known to cause skin rashes and discoloration of the skin during its acute stage. This condition usually affects people with weakened immune systems and those who are using improper medication on their bodies for a long time. The rashes may appear on different parts of your body, especially near the infected areas like the eyes or the genital areas. They are usually red in color but they can also be brownish in color or even yellowish in color based on how severe this infection is at the moment it is being treated.

Are the symptoms of Herpes the same for both men and women?

Both men and women have similar symptoms of herpes. Once you contract this disease, certain symptoms will follow. The initial symptoms of herpes are very mild, which is why it is important to note the causes, signs and symptoms of this disease.

Although some people do not experience any symptoms, other people may notice the following:

-Painful sores around the mouth or genital area

-Discharge from the penis in men / vagina in women

-Swollen lymph nodes in groin and neck area for several days

-Fever, headaches, muscle aches and tiredness.

How to avoid the spread of Herpes

Avoiding the spread of Herpes is one of the most important steps in reducing the severity and frequency of outbreaks.

The main way to avoid spreading herpes is to avoid direct skin contact with an active Herpes outbreak. In other words, don't have sex with an infected person when they are displaying active symptoms.

This can be difficult, because most people don't realize that they have been exposed! They may think, "I must have gotten it from my girlfriend last week, but she hasn't had any outbreaks since then... so I must be clear." But this person could still be spreading the virus without having any visible symptoms! So even if you were 100% sure that you contracted the virus from someone else – what if they were wrong? Or what if they just didn't remember? It is also important to keep in mind that the virus can be spread even when there are no visible symptoms.

It's best to avoid sex altogether, but if you do choose to have sex, use a condom every single time. Even if you trust your partner and are sexually monogamous, as the saying goes "better safe than sorry". Of course, in order for condoms to work properly they must be used correctly.

Although there is a slim chance to avoid an infection if you are unaware, make sure you know which symptoms to look out for so that you can stay informed. In fact, your partner should know what symptoms to look out for as well so that they can recognize and avoid outbreaks in the future.

Herpes and AIDS: Is there a relationship?

There has been much discussion over the years about a possible link between herpes virus and AIDS. There are some who think that both are caused by the same virus. Others believe that they are two distinct viruses, but one may be able to lead to the other. There are also some who believe that neither disease is caused by a virus at all and it is more of a dietary deficiency resulting in immune suppression. To date, there has been no proof of any connection between these two diseases.

However, it is known that being immune-suppressed does put people at risk for contracting any type of illness or virus, including herpes. AIDS patients with herpes have their outbreaks more frequently than people with AIDS and no herpes virus or even people who don't have AIDS but who have herpes breaks out at all times. This could be because the body's immune system is too weak to prevent the outbreak from occurring which shows how dangerous it can be to have an immune deficiency when dealing with any infection.

Another thing to consider is the fact that AIDS patients are given the antiviral drug acyclovir for herpes treatments. (Acyclovir is also used for shingles and chickenpox.) The drug was at first only tested on AIDS patients because there were no other options, but it was found to be effective in preventing outbreaks even in non-HIV patients. This could be because AIDS patients are known to have low levels of T-cells which is what makes up the immune system.

It has been proven that herpes virus can spread through sexual contact and blood transfusions. It also can be transferred from mother to child while in utero or during birth. Many researchers believe that it would not take much for a person with HIV or AIDS to contract genital herpes if intimate contact with someone who has an outbreak occurs.

Chapter 3

Who is Dr. Sebi?

Dr. Sebi is a renowned herbalist, a herbal doctor, and a healer. He was born in the small village of La Gomera, Honduras on November 26, 1933 and died on July 06, 2016. He left behind an extensive legacy of over 300 scientific and herbal research findings and books. The world has lost a great man, but his legacy lives on. He was one of the first to discover the connection between viruses and cancer. He is known around the world for curing people from cancer.

Dr. Sebi the herbalist

Dr. Sebi is the most sought after herbalist in the world. His herbal formulations have been effective in curing people of cancer, HIV / AIDS, diabetes, herpes, and other chronic diseases. **He is known for curing many celebrities including:** Lisa Bonet (actress), Michael Jackson (singer), Eddie Murphy (actor), Celia Cruz (singer), Steven Seagal (actor) and many others.

Dr. Sebi has formulated his herbal remedies in various ways: tinctures, capsules, ointments and topical solutions and only uses the highest quality ingredients. His herbal remedies are sold in many countries all over the world.

Science and herbs

Dr. Sebi uses the science of MicroBiology to cure herpes, which is very different from traditional medical practice. Traditional practice uses antiviral drugs, such as acyclovir, that are manufactured and distributed by drug companies. Dr. Sebi's method involves no drugs and no pharmaceutical companies.

Herbs are the basis of Dr. Sebi's method for curing herpes. He uses a combination of herbs that comes from one source; the African continent. Dr. Sebi has the ability to prepare the herbs in a way that enhances their healing properties and makes them much more effective than they would be as isolated single-herb products.

Dr. Sebi says that he uses his Microbiology knowledge to break down the virus", which is what creates this healing effect on herpes. This is very different from traditional medical practice, which uses antiviral drugs to treat herpes and other viruses. Antivirals are designed to attack viruses by preventing them from multiplying or attaching themselves to cells in your body (the way viruses spread). However, these synthetic drugs don't get rid of the virus entirely and eventually you will develop resistance to these pharmaceutical products, which will require you to take more drugs or a different drug altogether that the virus has not yet become resistant to. The side effects from antiviral drugs are also quite severe compared with those of herbs and other natural remedies for herpes like Dr. Sebi's recommended herbs.

The science behind the herbs in Dr. Sebi's Herpes cure is as follows:

1.Olive Leaf Extract

The olive tree is a symbol of fertility and peace. Olive leaves have been used for many years to cure bacterial infections like staphylococcus, streptococcus, and tuberculosis. Olive leaves contain the trace elements and minerals chromium, nickel, copper, zinc, cobalt, manganese, potassium, selenium, silicon and magnesium. These elements are essential in activating the immune system to destroy certain cells that could turn cancerous. Specifically the trace element chromium is used by the body to fight against viruses such as herpes and hepatitis. Olive leaf extract is also a natural antihistamine (meaning it will not cause sleepiness like Benadryl).

2.Oregano Extract

Oregano leaves contain carvacrol and thymol, both of which are antifungal and antibacterial. They have been used topically to treat skin infections, pneumonia, intestinal yeast infections, and vaginal yeast infections. Oregano leaves contain high amounts of thymus protein, which is the immune system's natural defense mechanism against bacteria and germs. Thymus protein has been known to increase white blood cell count.

3.Thyme Extract

Thyme used topically in small amounts can cure athlete's foot, ringworm, boils, infected wounds, acne, cold sores and insect bites. Thyme is a natural antibiotic that stimulates the immune system to fight against viruses like herpes. It also contains the same element chromium as olive leaf extract. Thyme inhibits virus replication by binding to the virus itself. This stops the virus from uncoiling itself so it cannot multiply or socially attach itself to other cells in the body in order to replicate itself (i.e., cause a cold sore).

Dr. Sebi recognizes the importance of a healthy diet and living in harmony with the earth's natural cycles. He believes that a healthy diet high in raw fruit and vegetable consumption, with an emphasis on organically grown produce, is essential to keeping the body free of illness.

Dr. Sebi's teachings on the power of herbs

Dr. Sebi's method to cure herpes is a simple one that involves oregano oil, garlic, and cayenne pepper as well as some other herbs.

The herpes virus is a tricky one that has been around since the beginning of time. It was passed from generation to generation and was a silent killer in which the person infected with the herpes virus could infect someone else without them knowing it. The only way you could know if you had the herpes virus was by testing yourself.

Dr. Sebi had patients come to his clinic with herpes who had no idea that they were infected. This is where Dr. Sebi would put his herbs to use in order to cure this disease that was plaguing humanity for so many years. Dr. Sebi's method of curing herpes involved many things, but mainly an herb called "Thyme" which Dr. Sebi used as a tea for his patients who had the herpes virus in their system, he would explain to them how this herb worked along with garlic and oregano oil; these three natural ingredients worked together to rid the body of the herpes virus while not harming any vital organs or fluids in your body at all, it simply killed off the virus and then disappeared completely from your body once it was gone, never to return again.

In addition, over the years, Dr. Sebi has formulated herbs and healing ingredients in the form of drinkable smoothies, making it easier to consume the herbs, especially for younger patients who do not have the time to sit down and drink a cup of tea. Dr. Sebi's method to cure herpes is perfect for anyone who wants to rid themselves of this disease once and for all without having to spend countless amounts of money on doctor bills, medications, or tests.

Chapter 4

Dr. Sebi's Method to Cure Herpes

Now that we have a clear understanding of who Dr. Sebi is, we will look at his teachings and how he healed thousands of people suffering from Herpes in particular.

In this chapter, you will learn how Dr. Sebi cured his own herpes as well as those of thousands of people who were affected by it.

Most people have been taught that there is no cure for herpes, but this is not true. The fact that you are reading this book means that you have probably tried many things to get rid of the virus already without any success. I have been there, and I know what it feels like to be stuck with a virus that you just can't get rid of no matter how many times you try.

After years of trying different methods to get rid of my herpes, I finally found something that worked. **The method was a combination of two distinct approaches:** Sebi's herbal treatment and Alkaline Diet. This combination produced results after just one month; however, it took me more than two years to put everything together and come up with a detailed plan on how to treat herpes naturally without having any side effects.

We will also explain the origins of the recommended treatment and how it has been used successfully by thousands of people.

One thing that you should know is that this treatment is not a quick fix. It's not a one-time shot or a magic pill that you take and you are cured.

This method is simple, but it will require your time and effort to complete; however, the results will be worth it. If you follow these steps diligently, you will be free from the herpes virus in a few months.

Allopathic Medicine is Not the Answer

Allopathic medicine tells people that they have to manage the symptoms of herpes. In other words, allopathic medicine treats the symptoms but not the disease itself.

Many people are afraid of trying alternative methods because they think it's too dangerous, but this shouldn't be your first thought. Most alternative treatments are safer than conventional medicines; in fact, many people have been cured by using herbal remedies alone.

Herbal remedies have been used for thousands of years for various medical conditions without any side effects and with amazing results. The problem is that most doctors are not aware of these remedies because they don't need to know about them in order to get a license or sell prescription drugs. It's funny, but the medical doctors don't want you to know about alternative medicine because they don't need it. But if your life's on the line, don't you think that you should have a better option than the one that is available?

You will find out more about herbal treatment in this chapter and how Dr. Sebi cured his own herpes as well as thousands of other people.

Given that the conventional method is failing to heal people, it's time to look for an alternative.

What Dr. Sebi Has Proven

Dr. Sebi had proven that the conventional treatment of herpes using prescription drugs is just a way to make money for pharmaceutical companies and not a cure for herpes. He also proved that he can treat people with herbal remedies only and achieve amazing results.

It is sad to say, but most people are not aware of the power of natural healing. Most people still believe that there is no cure for herpes and that it's the same disease that can never be fully healed.

The biggest problem in this situation is that most people don't take the required time to research a treatment in order to know if it's going to work for them or not.

Most of the time people are just looking for quick fixes, but this is not the way we should approach our health. Most people are looking for a magic pill or a one-time shot, but this doesn't exist. We have to remember that we cannot solve big problems with short-term solutions.

For example, if you want to lose weight, you cannot just go for a diet and exercise program for a week and expect to lose weight. This will work only in the short run because your body will return back to its original state once you stop exercising or reduce your diet. In order to achieve permanent results, you have to keep exercising after the diet ends and eat right forever.

The same applies when you are trying some alternative methods: if you try something for a week or two then quit, then your herpes will come back with a vengeance because your body didn't get enough time to heal completely from the inside out.

This is why you have to take the required time and make sure that you do everything right before you start to see results. It usually takes a few months or even years of hard work in order to completely heal from herpes; however, it is worth all the effort, and you will be amazed at the results.

How Dr. Sebi Found His Cure

Dr. Sebi is a healer and herbalist from Honduras who found a unique cure to herpes that was not available in the medical field, and he was able to prove that people can heal themselves through natural methods. He had observed that the people who lived in his country were healthy but still suffered from life-threatening diseases such as cancer and diabetes.

He also noticed that the people who traveled outside of their country to other countries were suffering from the same diseases which were common in those countries, but they did not have these diseases when they lived in their homeland.

This made Dr. Sebi question why there is such a difference between people living in different countries, and why do some of them get sick while others don't? His conclusion was that it is all about how we are treating our body inside out.

In order to truly heal yourself of herpes, you have to find what is making your body unhealthy and treat it before you can naturally cure your body of this virus. You have to make sure that your body has the right mix of all essential nutrients (vitamins, minerals) and then cleanse your liver because this will help you remove all toxins from your body faster than ever before. When you take care of the inside, the outside will take care of itself, so you will be free of herpes forever.

This is how Dr. Sebi found his cure for herpes that he used to heal thousands of people from this virus.

Dr. Sebi's Natural Process

1.Stop taking Prescription Drugs

The first step to curing herpes is to stop using drugs. In fact, you should never take any pharmaceutical drug for herpes, because these drugs will only slow down your progress and they also have side effects that are worse than the disease itself.

For example, most people think that taking prescription drugs is a good way to treat herpes, but this is not the case. Prescription drugs are not like vitamins or supplements. When you take a pharmaceutical drug, your body will perceive it as a poison, and it will try to get rid of this poison by flushing it through your liver into the toilet.

Because most drugs don't dissolve in water, they have to go through your liver first, and this process can take up to 2 weeks. During this time, your liver will be working on getting rid of the drug, and you will feel bad.

Moreover, most drugs can damage your liver. For instance, Valtrex is one of the most popular prescription drugs for herpes treatment; however, it has a side effect on the liver that can be deadly if you are not careful.

In fact, Valtrex can cause liver failure, and this is why you should never take it.

Another example of a prescription drug for herpes that can damage your liver is Aciclovir. Even though it's a natural drug, it can still cause damage to your liver; therefore, you should avoid taking this drug as well.

On the other hand, there is a natural way to heal yourself from herpes without any drugs or supplements. We will discuss this method further in the next chapter; however, you should know that you must stop taking prescription drugs before starting the natural process of healing from herpes. Otherwise, your body might prefer getting rid of the drugs and not work on healing itself.

2.Herpes Cleanse

In order to start the healing process, you must cleanse your body completely of all toxins. Toxins build up in your body over time, and this is why it's important to cleanse your body at least once a year. Once you have stopped taking drugs, you should take several days in order to cleanse your liver and colon.

You can do this by eating healthy foods like fresh vegetables and fruits. You can also try some colon cleansing methods in order to make sure that your body is clean of toxins.

3.Herpes Diet

After your body is clean, you should start the diet that Dr. Sebi recommends to his patients. The diet consists of eating fresh fruits, non-starchy vegetables, and baked chicken for three days at a time. During these three days, you should drink lots of purified water to flush out all toxins from your body.

The idea behind this diet is to severely limit carbohydrates and sugar intake from food in order to make your body burn fat instead of sugar for energy. This is a very beneficial way to lose weight because it burns fat from the inside out instead of just losing weight on the skin like most diets do; however, this method is not easy because it requires a lot of willpower.

For example, when you eat carbs and sugar it will give you a rush of energy which makes you feel good; therefore, most people find it difficult to go without carbs and sugar in their daily diets because they are addicted to them more than anything else. **It's like an addiction:** if you have been eating tacos or pizza every day for the last 20 years then it is going to be extremely difficult for you to stop eating them.

This is why you have to be very determined when you start this diet, because if you give up after a few days then you will never achieve the results that you want. Most people are not mentally prepared for this challenge, and they give up before they actually start seeing results.

The reason why most people fail on this diet is because of their emotional attachments to food. If you can remove your emotional ties with food then losing weight will be a piece of cake. In fact, it's not about losing weight, but about becoming healthy and staying that way for the rest of your life.

In order to help with your emotions and make sure that you continue with the diet, try not to eat in front of the television because it will make it harder for you to resist food cravings. For example, if you are watching your favorite television show while eating pizza or something else unhealthy, then it is going to make it harder for you to resist these foods; therefore, eat at least 30 minutes before watching television so that your mind focuses on something other than food. If you can do this then eating healthy will become your natural tendency and you will not be tempted to eat unhealthy foods because you will have something else to keep your mind occupied.

4.Herpes Juicing

In addition to eating healthy and drinking lots of water, you should also drink fresh vegetable juice that Dr. Sebi recommends in order to boost your immune system and cleanse your body completely from the inside out. However, you should never use a juicer in order to make juice because it is not powerful enough for this purpose; instead, you can use a blender or even a food processor. You can also buy fresh juice at some grocery stores; however, it is always better to make juice yourself because it is always 100% organic and free of any preservatives or chemicals.

Juicing is an important step for healing yourself from herpes because it helps your body get rid of toxins and chemicals which slow down the healing process. For example, most people think that eating healthy helps them stay healthy, but this is not true. Even if you eat only vegetables and fruits every day, your body will still contain toxins that are produced by stress or by the environment; therefore, it's important for you to cleanse your body completely with juices in order for your body to heal itself.

Chapter 5

Dr. Sebi's Herbs Used to Treat Herpes

Dr. Sebi has found that the ultimate cure for Herpes is the combination of his herbal remedies and a diet that consists of fresh organic fruits and vegetables. However, he has included in this book some other herbs that he uses in his herbal formula for herpes.

In this chapter, we will learn about the herbs that Dr. Sebi uses to treat herpes and how he combines them with other herbs to create a formula that gets results.

Herb that cures herpes naturally

Dr. Sebi believes that natural healing starts with a healthy gut. This is because the gut is connected to the immune system which is responsible for destroying invading pathogens such as viruses. Therefore, the first thing Dr. Sebi does when he is approached by people with herpes is to assess their overall health condition.

There are various herbs which allows the body to heal and these herbs are used to treat the herpes virus. These herbs are natural medicines that Dr. Sebi recommends for the treatment of herpes. **The herbs include:**

1.Black seed (Nigella sativa)

Dr. Sebi recommends black seed as an antiviral agent to treat herpes. Black seed has been used throughout history for various purposes. It is known for its antioxidant properties which makes it effective in treating various ailments including herpes. Studies have shown that black seed is effective in healing numerous skin conditions including fungal infections and acne.

2.Black sesame seed (Sesamum indicum)

Black sesame seed can be used to treat herpes and it has many other health benefits as well. The seeds are rich in polyunsaturated fats and amino acids and these nutrients are known to have anti-inflammatory properties. Black sesame seeds have been used for centuries in Asia as a natural treatment for various skin conditions including eczema, psoriasis, and even acne. In addition, black sesame seeds are rich sources of vitamins A, B1, B2, B3, B6, C, E and K as well as minerals such as iron, calcium, copper, zinc and magnesium among others. These nutrients help the body to get rid of the viral infection that causes herpes outbreak on your skin.

3.Olive leaf (Olea europaea)

Olive leaf is another herb which Dr Sebi recommends for treatment of the herpes virus. Olive leaf contains a compound called oleuropein which has been shown to have anti-inflammatory properties. This compound is also known to boost the immune system and kill the herpes virus. The powerful antiviral properties of olive leaf help to eliminate the herpes virus from your body.

4.Neem (Azadirachta indica)

Dr Sebi recommends neem for healing the skin of people with herpes as it has been used for treatment of various skin problems. Neem contains a compound called azadirachtin which is known to have powerful anti-viral properties. It is therefore effective in treating herpes as well as boosting immunity against this infection. It also contains other beneficial compounds such as terpenoids and limonoids which are known to have anti-inflammatory and antioxidant properties.

5.Cloves (Syzygium aromaticum)

Cloves are another herb which Dr Sebi recommends for treating herpes outbreak on your skin and they contain antiviral compounds such as eugenol, linalool, cineole, neral, methyl chavicol and eugenol acetate among others that help in killing the viral infection that causes the outbreak of the virus on your skin. The antiviral compounds in cloves can also be applied directly on the affected areas of the skin to help you get rid of herpes.

6.Garlic (Allium sativum)

Garlic is another herb which Dr Sebi recommends for treating herpes outbreak on your skin. It contains active compounds such as allicin and selenium that are known to have antiviral properties. In addition to being an antiviral agent, garlic has anti-inflammatory properties which help in treating herpes outbreaks and boost immunity against this viral infection. You can cut up a clove of garlic and apply it on the affected areas of the skin or you can drink a cup of garlic tea daily to boost your immunity against this viral infection.

7.Thyme (Thymus vulgaris)

Dr Sebi recommends thyme for treating herpes outbreak on your skin as it contains antiviral and antibacterial compounds that help in eliminating the virus from your system. Thyme is known to fight infections such as scabies, chicken pox, herpes, influenza colds, ringworms among others. The oils that are present in thyme have been used for centuries as a natural treatment for acne and eczema among other skin conditions including herpes.

8.Basil (Ocimum basilicum)

Basil contains antiviral compounds such as linalool, eugenol and methyl chavicol which are known to have potent anti-viral properties. It also contains cineole which is effective in treating skin conditions such as ringworms, chicken pox, mumps, measles and herpes among others. You can apply basil oil directly on the affected area of the skin or you can drink a cup of basil tea daily to boost your immunity against the viral infection that causes herpes outbreak on your skin.

9.Oregano (Origanum vulgare)

Dr Sebi recommends oregano for treating herpes outbreaks and it contains powerful phytochemicals including carvacrol that are known to have antiviral properties. This herb also contains thymol which is effective in treating infections such as herpes, mumps, chicken pox and measles among others. You can apply oregano oil directly on the affected areas of the skin or you can drink a cup of oregano tea daily. You may mix this herb with other herbs such as thyme to enhance their effectiveness in eliminating the virus from your body. Dr Sebi recommends taking oregano in combination with oregano oil rather than taking it raw.

10.Neem oil

Neem oil is another herb that Dr Sebi recommends for treating herpes outbreak on your skin as well as boosting your immunity against this viral infection. It contains compounds such as azadirachtin and limonoids which are known to have anti-inflammatory properties as well as being effective in eliminating the virus from your body. You may apply this oil directly on the affected areas of the skin or you can drink it in the form of neem tea to boost your immune response against this viral infection.

11.Tea tree (Melaleuca alternifolia)

Dr Sebi recommends tea trees for treating herpes outbreak on your skin and boosting immunity against this viral infection. This herb contains a compound called terpinen-4-ol that has been shown to have potent anti-viral properties and also has anti-inflammatory properties which help in treating herpes outbreaks on your skin. You can apply tea tree oil directly on the affected areas of the skin or you can drink a cup of tea tree tea daily to boost your immune system against this virus.

The Gourd antioxidant that fights off viruses

Gourd can be used in the treatment of herpes. Garlic, turmeric, cinnamon bark and olive oil can also be used in the treatment of herpes. These herbs are potent antioxidants that fight off viruses and bacteria.

Dr. Sebi's gourd was the cure for many of the viruses and bacteria that were attacking his patients. Dr. Sebi uses gourd seeds (also known as calabash or bottle gourds) which are very high in antioxidants and an amazing source of vitamins, minerals, anti-oxidants, and essential fatty acids. Dr. Sebi used the entire fruit and the seeds in his herbal medicines. The seeds are very high in vitamins A, B1, B2, B3, B6, C and E.

Vitamins A and C are best known for their anti-viral properties. Vitamin C is also a powerful antioxidant that neutralizes free radicals (bad oxygen molecules). Vitamin A is also an antioxidant that helps heal viral infections by supporting the immune system. Both of these vitamins are essential for a healthy immune system that fights off viruses and bacteria. Eaten raw or juiced, the gourd seed's vitamin content stays intact due to their high fiber levels which help to cleanse the body of toxins while absorbing water from the digestive tract to create a large volume of bulky stools with healthy kidney-friendly electrolytes (like potassium) which help to flush out bad toxins from your body.

Gourd seed soup:

Gourd seeds provide high amounts of fiber and protein as well as minerals such as beta-carotene (which is converted into vitamin A), zinc and calcium; all essential nutrients for good health or for healing on any level – physically, emotionally, mentally or spiritually.

Gourd seeds have anti-inflammatory properties that are essential for fighting off viruses and bacteria and therefore help to heal ailments such as herpes. Flax seeds, pumpkin seeds and sesame seeds are other high fiber foods that are also anti-inflammatory. Anti-inflammatory foods help to reduce swelling in the body and the throat which helps to heal herpes sores on a physical level. Reducing inflammation in your body will also help to ease feelings of anger, resentment, frustration or fear which can spark outbreaks of herpes or other viral infections.

The gourd seed is an excellent source of protein for healing herpes. Protein is the nutrient that helps to rebuild cells on a cellular level (including cell walls). Eating more protein will help you feel more energetic while rebuilding your immune system so that it is better able to fight off viruses and bacteria – including herpes! Foods high in protein include fish (salmon, mackerel, sardines), chicken (wings, legs), beef (brisket, chuck roast), lamb (legs), pork (legs, loin) and gourd seeds. You may also want to try any of Dr. Sebi's Sebi Protein Powders.

The gourd seed is also very high in beta-carotene which the body converts into vitamin A. Vitamin A is essential for rebuilding skin tissue on a cellular level and for fighting off viruses and bacteria. However, too much vitamin A can be toxic to the body so it's important to get a balanced amount of vitamin A from a variety of foods rather than relying on supplements containing excessive vitamin A. Foods high in beta-carotene include carrots, bell peppers, spinach, kale, cauliflower and cantaloupe.

Dandelion and its abilities

Dandelion is an herb that is native to Europe but has spread to the Americas, to the Far East and Australia. Dandelion is a perennial plant that grows in most parts of the world. The dandelion plant has flowers in yellow or white colors, which bloom during the summer season. Dandelion leaves are dark green and jagged with finger-like projections. The roots of dandelion plants are yellow-white colored with a brownish center.

Dr. Sebi recommends the use of dandelion to treat herpes. Dandelion is one of the most effective natural herbs that is used in a number of remedies. It helps to stimulate the liver, which in turn flushes out toxic matter and aids in the removal of all kinds of viruses. Dandelion is also good for detoxifying the liver and the blood.

Dandelion has a bitter taste, which makes it perfect for cleansing the liver. Dandelion is also rich in vitamins A, B1, B2, C and K. This herb is also rich in potassium, calcium and magnesium. The dandelion herb helps to cleanse the kidneys and gallbladder while ridding your body of toxins.

As a treatment for Herpes, dandelion is one of the best herbs. Dandelion leaves and roots are used in preparing a number of tonics and remedies. The dandelion leaves can also be used as a salad as well as used in soups. Dandelion leaves are rich in vitamins A, B1, B2, C and K. They are also rich in iron, calcium, magnesium and potassium.

The dandelion roots have a number of healing properties that make it perfect for treating Herpes infections. The dandelion root contains vitamin B complex, which includes vitamins A, B1 and B2. Dandelion also contains vitamin C that helps to fight against colds and flus. This herb is also rich in zinc that helps to get rid of Herpes virus infections from the body system.

In addition to being able to get rid of Herpes virus from your body system, the dandelion herb can be used on its own with other herbs to treat this viral infection. The dandelion herb helps in triggering the liver cells to flush out toxins in the body thereby helping you clear out Herpes virus from your body system. It likewise assists with getting rid of scar tissues created by the disease from your body system. It also helps in the removal of Herpes virus from your body system.

In addition to helping with the removal of Herpes virus from your body system, dandelion also helps in improving the immune system. Dandelion is therefore a good herb for fighting against colds, flues and other cardiovascular diseases.

Using Basil to fight herpes

Basil is a herb that can be used in different ways to treat Herpes. Basil is a small plant that belongs to the family of mints. This herb has small leaves and tiny white flowers. The basil plant grows well in most parts of the world. It can be grown indoors and outdoors.

The basil plant is one of the most popular herbs in all parts of the world. It is used as a culinary herb and also for preparing drinks and medicines for treating colds, flus, stomach aches, infections and other diseases. The basil leaves have medicinal properties that help to fight against many diseases including Herpes virus infections.

Basil leaves are rich in vitamins A, B1, B2, C and K as well as calcium, magnesium and iron. These herbs are also good for fighting against colds, flues and other cardiovascular diseases. The basil leaves have anti inflammatory properties that help to relieve pain caused by Herpes virus infection from your body system as well as speeding up healing of this disease from your body system.

When using Basil to treat Herpes infections you should make sure that you only use fresh basil leaves since they contain more medicinal properties than dried ones do.

Using Lavender to fight herpes

Lavender is one of the most important natural herbs that are used in fighting against Herpes virus. The lavender plant has a fresh smell and a bright purple color. Lavender flowers are usually used in making essential oils aimed at treating infections such as Herpes virus.

The lavender herb has been used for a long time as an antiseptic agent. In addition, it is also commonly used to treat wounds and sores. Lavender oil is also used by many people to treat depression, insomnia, anxiety and stress among other health conditions.

Lavender has several healing properties that makes it perfect for treating herpes infections in the body system. In addition to being able to help with the treatment of Herpes virus infections in your body system, the lavender herb is also good for treating skin conditions such as burns, cuts and rashes. This herb can be used on its own or with other herbs to treat Herpes viral infections in your body system. In fact, it works best when combined with other herbs such as dandelion root, cayenne pepper extract among others.

Olive Leaf and its efficiency

Olive leaf is a very powerful natural remedy that has been used for curing all kinds of viruses and bacteria infections in the body system. The olive leaf herb contains a number of vitamins and minerals including vitamins A, B1, B2, C and K. Olive leaves are rich in iron, calcium, phosphorus and potassium.

Olive Leaf Extract is also rich in antioxidants that help to fight against free radicals in the body system. This herb helps to boost the immune system while at the same time boosting your body's overall health. Olive leaf extract is also used in fighting against Herpes virus infections since it helps to inhibit viral replication thereby rendering the viral infection unable to spread from one cell to another.

In addition to helping with ridding your body of Herpes virus infections, olive leaves are also used for treating colds and flues since they have a number of antioxidants that help to boost the immune system while at the same time boosting your overall health.

Olive Leaves have a bitter taste, which makes it one of the most effective herbs when it comes to fighting off all kinds of bacteria and viruses from your body system. Olive leaf extract can be taken as tea or as tinctures mixed with honey. You can also use olive leaf extract as a compound for preparing other herbal remedies that help in getting rid of Herpes virus infections from your body system.

Chapter 6

The Dr. Sebi Diet for Herpes

The Dr. Sebi diet for herpes is very simple to follow. There are three simple food groups that we must eat on a regular basis in order to eliminate herpes from our bodies. **The three food groups are:**

Vegetables: We must eat a minimum of four cups of vegetables daily. The vegetables should be fresh and uncooked. They should never be canned, frozen, or cooked in any other way. **The best vegetables are:** carrots, yams, celery, squash, cabbage and broccoli. **Grains:** We must eat two to three cups of uncooked grains each day. The best grains are quinoa, amaranth and oats (not the instant kind). **Fruits:** We must eat a minimum of two cups of fresh fruits each day. The best fruits are bananas, strawberries and cantaloupe (not the juice).

When we combine these three food groups each day, our bodies will produce powerful enzymes that will kill all the viruses in our systems!

Drinking Water: We must drink a minimum of six glasses of water each day to help cleanse our systems of impurities that may be causing us to get herpes. Water is also very important to our overall health and well-being. The best water to drink is distilled water.

Supplements: Supplements are very important for the Dr. Sebi diet for herpes. They help us quickly detoxify our bodies and fight off any viruses that we may encounter during the day. **There are many different supplements that we can take, but the best ones for this diet are:** oregano oil capsules, olive leaf extract, beet root powder, probiotics and vitamin C. You can purchase all of these supplements at any health food store or online.

Why a Proper Diet Is Paramount for Herpes

In order to properly understand why a proper diet is paramount for herpes, we must first understand what causes the virus to live in our bodies. The virus does not live on any food that we eat. It lives within our body cells and is protected by the cell membranes. We can eat all of the foods that we want and this will not eliminate the virus from our bodies. In order to eliminate the virus, we must follow a diet that will cause a powerful reaction within our bodies. When we eat foods that make us sick, such as sugars, fats and animal products, it weakens our immune systems and allows for viruses such as herpes to enter our systems. When we eat fresh fruits and vegetables (especially juicing them), it makes us feel healthy and strong so that the viruses will have no chance of gaining control over us.

The body cells that harbor the virus must be eliminated by the body to eliminate the virus. Cells are constantly being created and eliminated by our bodies, so it is not necessary to eliminate all of the cells in our bodies; but we do need to eliminate the cells that harbor viruses such as herpes. We do this by flushing our systems out through the elimination of old fecal matter and other bodily waste products. As a result, we will have healthy cell membranes in our bodies, which will prevent any foreign substances from entering into our systems; and will also prevent any viruses from multiplying within our bodies.

Having the proper diet will allow us to have the proper strength and energy, which is necessary for our immune systems to function properly. We will also have bright red blood cells, which will allow for proper oxygenation of our bodies. Cells that harbor viruses must be eliminated by our immune systems in order for us to be healthy and have a strong immune system.

As we eat more fresh fruits and vegetables, we are strengthening our immune systems and eliminating the pathogens that cause sickness and disease; thus eliminating the virus from our bodies. This is why a proper diet is paramount for herpes.

Fresh Fruits, Vegetables, Juices & Herbs:

The healing foods that will cure herpes are fresh fruits, vegetables and juices made from them. These are known as live foods because these foods contain enzymes that are alive in the bodies of those who consume them. These live enzymes help to strengthen the immune systems of those who eat them; thus allowing their body cells to become stronger so that they can fight off viruses such as herpes like a champ!

Drinking fresh vegetable juices made from carrots, apples, cucumbers & tomatoes (with celery if you can stand it) will flush out your intestinal lining much faster than eating whole fruits or vegetables by themselves. The reason for this is because your body will be able to absorb the nutrients in the juices quicker than it can digest whole fruits and vegetables. And since these juices do not contain any fiber, your body can easily eliminate them through your intestines and colon, thus flushing out toxins faster. (**Note:** These are not regular vegetable juices – they must be freshly made; and you must drink them on an empty stomach.)

These healing foods contain enzymes that help to strengthen our bodies and increase our energy levels. When we eat foods that contain live enzymes, it gives us energy to get up and go; whereas, eating dead foods makes us feel tired and sluggish because they deplete our energy levels by causing us to gain weight. Dead foods also cause constipation because they do not contain any fiber; whereas, live foods line our digestive tracts with fiber so that toxins can pass through our intestines faster.

Fresh fruits & vegetables help to flush out old fecal matter from our intestines & colons; which improves bowel movements, lowers blood pressure, helps us lose unwanted weight and increases the efficiency of our immune systems. People who don't eat enough fresh fruits & vegetables are usually constipated because they have old fecal matter lodged in their intestinal tracts. This old fecal matter is full of harmful bacteria, which is why we must flush our systems out as much as possible by eating plenty of fresh fruits & vegetables.

Herbs such as garlic, hot peppers, ginger, onions and turmeric will also help to cleanse our bodies from the harmful bacteria that causes many diseases. These herbs will also help to strengthen our immune systems and fight off viruses such as herpes.

The Diet for Herpes

1.Avoid all processed foods and dairy products.

Firstly, Dr. Sebi says, you should avoid all processed foods and dairy products. These foods are low-quality foods made from unhealthy sources. For example, processed foods are made from corn or wheat, which have been altered in some way to create a more desirable product. This process of altering the food lowers the quality of the food and also makes it a highly addictive substance.

Dairy products are not healthy for you because they are derived from cow's milk. Dr. Sebi says that cow's milk is not a natural food for humans because humans are the only mammals that consume the milk of another animal. There are also many health benefits to avoiding dairy products.

The body will not respond well to these foods because they are processed and have little or no nutritional value. Instead, you should eat whole, organic foods that are harvested from the ground.

Dr. Sebi recommends that you eat organic and fresh foods that are harvested from the ground.

2.Eat foods that are alkaline forming.

The next thing you need to do is eat foods that are alkaline-forming. The human body is naturally alkaline, which means that it should be slightly acidic. Achieving a pH balance of 7.365—which is slightly acidic—is critical for optimal health. However, the Western diet consists of many acidic foods, such as meats and dairy products.

Eating alkaline-forming foods will create an alkaline environment in the blood and muscles, which will kill off the virus causing herpes while maintaining the health of the infected area. Some of these foods include watermelon, papaya, cantaloupe, pineapple, grapefruit and blueberries.

The reason these foods are alkaline is because they contain nutrients that can neutralize acids in the body. To make sure that you are eating the right foods, you should consult a nutritionist.

3.Drink plenty of water.

Drinking plenty of water is very important in the healing process because it will flush out the infected blood cells and create an alkaline environment in the body. You should aim to drink at least two liters of water every day, and more if you are physically active.

4.Avoid all artificial sweeteners and refined sugar.

Artificial sweeteners are also acidic, so it is important to avoid them. If you have been drinking sodas or other sweetened drinks, you should slowly wean yourself off these products by replacing them with fresh fruit juices.

Refined sugar is another acidic food that can cause a viral infection in the body to multiply and spread. You should eliminate refined sugar from your diet and replace it with natural sugars such as honey, molasses, and maple syrup.

5.Eat plenty of vegetables and fruit.

Vegetables and fruit are also important parts of the diet because they contain antioxidants that help to flush out any viruses in the body while providing all the necessary nutrients for healing. Dr. Sebi also recommends that you eat plenty of raw foods like salads and fresh juice every day, which will help to flush out any viral cells in your bloodstream.

6.Eat unprocessed meats that are free-range, organic, or grass-fed.

Dr. Sebi says that beef is one of the best foods for healing herpes because it contains essential amino acids that stimulate the immune system while cleansing the blood stream of viruses and bacteria. Although most meats are acidic (which is why some people develop acid reflux when eating meat), grass-fed beef is alkaline.

Another benefit of eating beef is that it contains lysine, which is an amino acid that kills viruses in the body. You should also eat lamb and bison, which are also good sources of lysine. You should avoid processed meats like hot dogs and bacon because they are made from unhealthy ingredients.

7.Eat raw or cooked vegetables and fruits.

If you want to eat cooked vegetables, they should be lightly steamed to limit their exposure to heat and retain their nutritional value as much as possible. You should avoid microwaves because they destroy nutrients in the food. If you want to eat vegetables raw, make sure that you properly wash them so you do not become ill from bacteria and parasites.

8.Eat nuts, seeds, and legumes.

You should also eat nuts, seeds, and legumes because they are all alkaline-forming foods that stimulate the immune system. You should avoid peanuts because they contain mold and are not healthy for consumption.

9.Avoid all synthetic drugs and medications.

It is also important to avoid synthetic drugs and medications because they cause the body to become acidic. Many of these drugs cause a person to become depressed or lethargic, which can lead to an increase in viral activity within the body. You should only take natural herbs or supplements that have been prescribed by a doctor.

10.Eat foods that are low in hydrogenated oils or fats.

Dr. Sebi says that you should not eat foods that have been altered by hydrogenation because they contain trans fats, which are highly acidic and will make the body more prone to infection. To avoid trans fats, you should only eat foods that are unaltered by hydrogenation or other chemical processes.

11.Avoid all artificial additives and preservatives.

As with trans fats, you should avoid artificial additives in your diet because they can promote viral infections in the body while also causing a variety of health issues including cancer and diabetes. Some artificial additives include sodium benzoate, monosodium glutamate (MSG), aspartame, and saccharin. Make sure you read the labels on any food products before you buy them so you know what ingredients they contain.

12.Avoid all processed foods, fast foods, and junk foods.

You should also avoid processed foods, fast foods, and junk foods because they are low in nutrients and promote the growth of viral infections in the body. Many people purchase these products because they are affordable or convenient, but they do not provide your body with the nutrients it needs to fight off a viral infection. You should replace these products with whole, organic food sources that are harvested from the ground.

Dr. Sebi's Herpes Diet Plan

1.The diet must be followed for at least three months.

In order for the body to heal, the diet must be followed for a minimum of three months. When you begin to eat correctly, you will notice that things will get worse before they get better.

In other words, when you start eating right, your body begins to purge and this is what makes you feel worse. At the beginning of this process, you may feel achy all over and may have headaches (these are symptoms of the body purging), but after three months things will start getting better.

This process is sometimes called the "healing crisis" and it is a necessary process in order for the body to heal. The most important thing to do is not to give up!

For example, if you have been eating a lot of salty foods and your body has become accustomed to that type of diet, once you begin eating correctly you will experience achy joints, headaches, etc. During this healing crisis, the body is purging all the excess salt and toxins from the tissues.

This process can last for several months and this is why you must be patient with yourself and your diet. You must also understand that giving up on your new diet will only prolong this healing process.

So many people give up because they didn't realize that their bodies needed time to adjust to the change in diet. This is why I recommend following my plan for at least three to six months before giving up hope on it. It's just not that simple to change your life habits in one day.

The bottom line is: if you follow my plan correctly, it will work for you regardless of how long it takes for you to feel better. If you quit too soon, you won't get any results at all! Just be patient and stick with it until it starts working for you!

2.The diet must be followed strictly.

You need to eliminate all processed foods, sugars, starches, alcohol, dairy products and any other foods that don't agree with your body. Your diet should consist of fresh fruits (especially citrus), vegetables and high quality proteins such as organic eggs, chicken breast and fish.

3.You must take supplements to get rid of the virus and heal your body.

Most people who have herpes don't even realize that they have Candida or yeast overgrowth in their bodies along with the virus. Yeast feeds on sugar so if you have a yeast infection it means that you have been eating too many sugars and carbohydrates for your body to handle.

In order to completely heal from herpes you must eliminate Candida in your system, which means you must change your diet! Eliminating sugars, grains and starches will help starve the yeast infection in your body which will give you relief from painful outbreaks.

The best way to get rid of the yeast in your body is by taking a high quality anti-fungal supplement such as grapefruit seed extract. This natural anti-fungal has been used for years to treat Candida and other yeast related infections.

You can also add fresh garlic and colloidal silver to your diet to help boost your immune system and fight off viruses. In addition, I recommend taking a high quality probiotic supplement as well to help balance out your gut flora which is very important for overall health and well being.

4.Be careful not to overeat!

The key to healing from herpes with my diet is to eat only when you are hungry! Many people who have herpes are overweight because they eat too much food at one time and then they wonder why they have more outbreaks than anyone else! You must understand that eating too much food at one time goes against the body's natural rhythm and it will only stress the digestive system which can trigger an outbreak in some people. It is best if you eat every few hours, but make sure the meals are small in quantity; otherwise, you may over-stress your digestive organs which can weaken them over time.

5.You must avoid all stress!

Stress is a big contributor to outbreaks and I don't think that many people realize this. Stress is like poison to the body and it can weaken the immune system over time. If you are constantly feeling stressed out, then you must do something about it in order to heal from herpes!

The best way to reduce stress is by taking a few deep breaths throughout the day and making sure that you get plenty of sleep every night. It's also important to take some time each day to meditate and relax with your thoughts. Don't forget that laughter is also a great way to relieve stress, so make sure you have fun daily!

6.Be patient and give your body time to heal!

If you follow my diet plan correctly, it will work for your body regardless of how long it takes for you to feel better. Many people who come down with herpes are very stressed out about their situation which makes things worse for them; they become depressed and they begin eating more sugar just because they want comfort in their lives. This only makes things worse for them because they are adding more fuel (sugar) into an already raging fire (herpes virus)!

Conclusion

The information in this book is valuable and must be read by anyone who wants to understand how to cure herpes naturally. The methods that were explained here have worked for Dr. Sebi and anyone else who has been cured of herpes. Not only did they get rid of their herpes, but also their other medical conditions were addressed in the process.

Dr. Sebi was a natural healer who discovered that he could cure even the deadliest diseases with herbs. Herpes is also one of those diseases that Dr. Sebi was able to cure by using his herbs.

Dr. Sebi's Herpes Cure is a very powerful herbal treatment that does not only help you eliminate herpes, but also helps in dissolving and removing all types of cancerous cells from your body. Dr. Sebi's Herpes Cure does not only treat herpes, but eliminates it at its root.

This powerful herbal treatment is one of the best testimonies of this kind and it is very effective. It also helps in restoring the health of the body by getting rid of all kinds of infections and also helps in improving the immune system.

By learning how Dr. Sebi was able to cure himself of a slew of diseases and ailments and how he was able to get rid of different viruses from his body, you too can learn how to cure yourself from your condition. Just follow the steps that are laid out in this book and you will be able to get rid of all your ailments and diseases, especially for herpes.

As the saying goes, "knowledge is power." When you have the knowledge of how to cure yourself, you will be able to use this knowledge to change your life for the better. This book is a valuable resource for anyone who wants to learn how to cure herpes naturally.

If you are ready to stop living with herpes and start living a healthy life, then follow the teachings in this book and you will be able to do this. It is time for you to take control of your health, and Dr. Sebi has provided the necessary tools for you to do so.

You have everything that you need at your disposal; it is just up to you whether or not use it. Don't let herpes control your life any longer; instead, take charge of your health and live a healthier happier life today!

Herpes is not a death sentence. You can live a long and healthy life, but it is up to you if you want to achieve this.

We hope that you were able to learn many things from this book, and that you will use what you learned in this book to improve your health and your life.

Thank You

Thank you for buying my book and I hope you enjoyed it. If you found any value in this book I would really appreciate it if you'd take a minute to post a review about this book. I check all my reviews and love to get feedback.

Other Books By Author

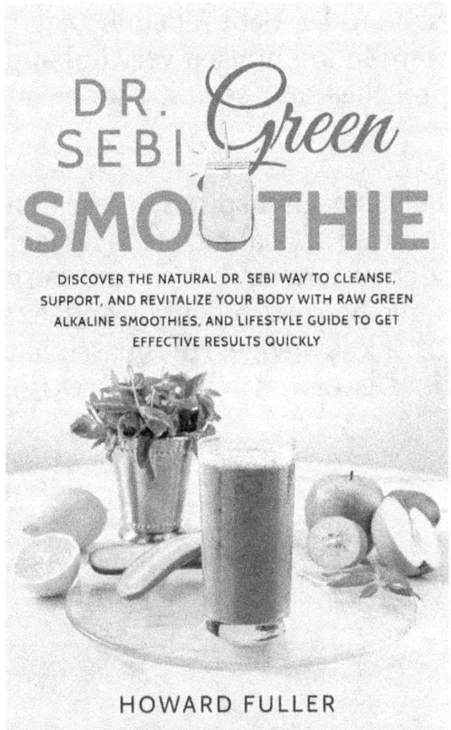

Dr. Sebi Green Smoothie:

Discover the Natural Dr. Sebi Way to Cleanse, Support, and Revitalize Your Body with Raw Green Alkaline Smoothies, and Lifestyle Guide to Get Effective Results Quickly

About Author

Howard Fuller is a college dietitian graduate who was healed from diabetes and high blood pressure after changing his dietary lifestyle to Dr. Sebi Alkaline Diet. Over the years in his career, Howard found himself very unhappy by one size fits all dietary approaches and seemingly one way road towards curing diseases.

Since then, he has been inspired to research and write about Dr. Sebi's natural way of healing. He loves cooking and writing about the wonder of natural health and herbal remedies. He has written many books deepening and expanding what is already a wealth of knowledge. He is passionate and truly loves what he does and is driven by the success he has of helping others achieve.